LOW SALT DIET FOR SENIORS

Comprehensive Guide to Reducing Sodium in Your Diet for Healthy Kidney and Heart Health.

Anita Pretzel

TABLE OF CONTENTS

INTRODUCTION 7

Chapter One 10

Understanding the Importance of a Low Salt Diet10

Introduction to Sodium and Its Impact on Senior Health 10

Risks Associated with High Sodium Intake in Seniors 12

Benefits of Adopting a Low Salt Diet for Senior Well-being 14

Chapter Two 17

Assessing Individual Sodium Needs for Seniors ..17

Determining Recommended Daily Sodium Intake for Seniors...17

Factors Influencing Sodium Requirements in Aging Individuals...19

Consulting with Healthcare Professionals for Personalized Guidance 21

Chapter Three 25

Identifying Hidden Sodium in Daily Foods 25

Uncovering Sneaky Sources of Salt in Common Foods 25

Reading Food Labels Effectively for Sodium Content 27

Cooking and Meal Preparation Tips for Minimizing Hidden Sodium..29

Chapter Four **33**

Creating a Flavorful Low Salt Diet Plan 33

Exploring Alternative Seasonings and Herbs 33

Cooking Techniques to Enhance Flavor Without Adding Salt...36

Sample Meal Plans Tailored for Seniors 40

Chapter Five **50**

Practical Tips for Dining Out on a Low Salt Diet ..50

Navigating Restaurant Menus for Low Sodium Options 50

Communicating Dietary Restrictions to Restaurant Staff...53

Enjoying Social Gatherings While Maintaining a Low Salt Lifestyle...57

Chapter Six...**61**

Managing Health Conditions with a Low Salt Diet61

Impact of Sodium Reduction on Hypertension and Cardiovascular Health.....................................61

Dietary Approaches for Seniors with Kidney Concerns 64

Collaborating with Healthcare Providers for Optimal Health Management.................................68

Chapter Seven 73

Overcoming Challenges and Resistance to a Low Salt Lifestyle 73

Addressing Common Concerns and Misconceptions 73

Strategies for Encouraging Family and Friends' Support 77

Motivational Techniques for Maintaining Long-Term Dietary Changes 81

Chapter Eight 85

Monitoring Sodium Intake and Tracking Progress85

Establishing a System for Tracking Daily Sodium Consumption...85

Recognizing and Celebrating Milestones in Salt Reduction 88

Adjusting the Diet Plan as Needed Based on Individual Responses 92

Chapter Nine **96**

Integrating Physical Activity and Lifestyle Choices96

Exploring the Connection Between Exercise and Sodium Balance 96

Incorporating Senior-Friendly Physical Activities....100

Holistic Approaches to Enhance Overall Well-being for Seniors 103

Conclusion...**107**

INTRODUCTION

Seniors' health becomes a top priority when their golden years draw to an end. Dietary decisions, especially the significance of sodium intake, are an important factor that is frequently disregarded yet has a significant impact. With an emphasis on the advantages and tactics catered specifically to the requirements of the elderly, The Low Salt Diet for Seniors provides a thorough road map to assist in navigating the challenging landscape of nutritional wellness.

This comprehensive book explores the complex relationship between salt and the health of older adults, as well as the dangers of consuming too much of it. It emphasizes the value of individualized strategies advised by medical professionals and gives users the expertise to evaluate their own salt demands.

Chapter 3 reveals the hidden sources of salt in common foods and offers helpful advice on how to read product labels and cook with awareness. The next chapter turns the low-sodium diet myth from tasteless to delectable by providing a variety of substitute herbs and seasonings as well as mouthwatering meals designed with elderly citizens in mind.

The difficulties that come with eating out are discussed in Chapter 5, where readers learn how to understand restaurant menus, explain dietary limitations, and enjoy social events without sacrificing their health objectives. Chapter 6 examines the effects of reducing salt on hypertension, cardiovascular health, and renal issues, promoting a cooperative approach with healthcare providers because health conditions and dietary decisions are frequently intertwined.

Chapter 7 discusses overcoming obstacles and resistance, addressing frequent worries, and offering inspiring tactics for sustained achievement. In Chapter 8, the guide emphasizes self-monitoring and progress tracking to make sure that changes are made as necessary for long-lasting beneficial results.

Lastly, by including lifestyle decisions and physical activity into the story, Chapter 9 widens the viewpoint. By acknowledging the relationship between diet and general health, elders can adopt holistic methods for a longer, happier life by reading this chapter.

Come along on this life-changing trip as we explore the subtleties of the Low Salt Diet for Seniors, a plan created to promote improved health, vigor, and longevity through lifestyle modifications as well as dietary adjustments.

CHAPTER ONE

UNDERSTANDING THE IMPORTANCE OF A LOW SALT DIET

Introduction to Sodium and Its Impact on Senior Health

The significance of making thoughtful and well-informed health decisions becomes more apparent as one approaches the end of their life. The importance of salt, an ingredient in our diets that seems to be present in everything yet is frequently underappreciated, takes center stage among the various aspects of senior well-being. The key to understanding the significant effects of salt on the health of older adults is provided by this introduction.

Sodium is a vital mineral that is important for many different body processes. But as we get older, keeping the right balance of salt becomes essential to good health. This chapter takes us on a trip to understand the complex relationship between sodium and older people's health.

We examine the physiological importance of sodium and how it affects neuronal transmission, muscle contractions, and fluid balance. At the same time, we have to face the harsh truth that elderly people's health can be seriously jeopardized by consuming excessive amounts of salt. Elevated salt levels have long-term negative impacts on the aging process, ranging from hypertension to cardiovascular problems.

As we explore the subtleties of sodium metabolism in the elderly, we also highlight the sometimes disregarded link between sodium and prevalent health issues that older people encounter. The goal is to empower elders by providing them with the knowledge base they need to make educated food decisions, rather than to engender dread.

This chapter lays the foundation for a deeper investigation of the effects of sodium on the health of older adults. It also covers hidden sources of salt, customized sodium demands, and doable tactics for adopting a low-sodium lifestyle. Let's travel the sodium spectrum together with clarity, compassion, and a dedication to promoting a more vibrant, healthy trip through old age.

Risks Associated with High Sodium Intake in Seniors

The influence of food decisions on senior health is felt more and more as the golden years pass. Sodium is one of the dietary culprits that should be carefully considered because it may indicate health problems if ingested in excess. In this chapter, we explore the particular hazards connected to high sodium intake in the elderly, providing insight into the complexities of this sometimes-disregarded health issue.

1. Hypertension and Cardiovascular Complications: Examining the relationship between high sodium intake and hypertension, a common issue among the elderly

deciphering the cascade effect, which explains how cardiovascular issues like heart disease and stroke are exacerbated by hypertension.

2. Fluid Retention and Edema: Examining how sodium affects fluid balance and whether too much sodium might cause fluid retention

recognizing the ways in which edema, a symptom of fluid retention, affects elderly people's movement and comfort in general.

3. Renal Strain and Kidney Concerns: Analyzing the complex connection between high sodium consumption and kidney function in the elderly

emphasizing the dangers of renal strain, such as the emergence or aggravation of kidney-related problems.

4. Implications for Cognitive Function: Examining recent findings about the relationship between salt levels and aging-related cognitive impairment

discussing how a high-salt diet may exacerbate diseases like dementia and Alzheimer's disease.

5. Bone Health and Osteoporosis: Examining the relationship between senior bone density, calcium, and sodium

Exposing the possible links between elevated sodium levels and osteoporosis and weakened bone structure

6. Increased Risk of Dehydration: talking about how too much sodium can cause dehydration, which is especially important for seniors who may already be more susceptible to the condition.

Benefits of Adopting a Low Salt Diet for Senior Well-being

When it comes to achieving bright health in your golden years, food decisions become invaluable allies. A low-salt diet stands out as a revolutionary strategy with numerous advantages as seniors negotiate the complex world of nutrition. This chapter examines the benefits and all-around advantages that adopting a low-salt lifestyle can have for senior citizens' health.

1. Blood Pressure Management: Explaining how eating a low-salt diet helps to keep blood pressure levels in check

examining the possibility of lowering the risk of hypertension and related cardiovascular problems.

2. Cardiovascular Health: Looking into how consuming less sodium can improve heart health in general.

talking about how a low-sodium diet may help reduce the risk of stroke and heart disease.

3. Enhanced Fluid Balance: Learning how the body's ideal fluid balance is promoted by a low-salt diet

investigating the possibility of less fluid retention and the discomfort that comes with it.

4. Kidney Function Support: talking about how a low-salt diet might help relieve kidney strain.

investigating the potential benefits of lower sodium consumption for renal function and health.

5. Cognitive Well-Being: Examining recent findings regarding the relationship between salt levels and mental well-being

talking about how a low-sodium diet may help maintain brain health and lower the chance of cognitive decline.

6. Bone Health Preservation: Examining the potential benefits of a low-salt diet for maintaining bone density

talking about the possible advantages of promoting general skeletal health and lowering the risk of osteoporosis.

7. Better Hydration: Stressing the benefits of a low-salt diet on improved hydration

encouraging seniors who are susceptible to dehydration to talk about the value of maintaining appropriate hydration.

8. Weight Management: Examining how a low-sodium diet may help seniors control their weight talking about how consuming less sodium might help you keep a healthy weight.

CHAPTER TWO

ASSESSING INDIVIDUAL SODIUM NEEDS FOR SENIORS

Determining Recommended Daily Sodium Intake for Seniors

A vital factor to take into account when seniors set out to optimize their health is knowing how much sodium they should consume each day and adjusting it to suit their individual requirements. This chapter examines the complex process of figuring out how much salt should be consumed daily by seniors, taking into account their unique dietary needs and the effect it has on their general health.

1. Knowing Baseline Sodium Recommendations: Examining accepted recommendations for sodium consumption in general and how they relate to older citizens

talking about the reasoning behind the health authorities' daily salt recommendations.

2. Factors Affecting Senior Sodium Needs: Understanding the distinct physiological alterations that come with aging and how they affect the metabolism of sodium going over how different things like kidney function, drugs, and general health might affect a person's demand for sodium.

3. Individualized Methods with Medical Experts:

stressing the value of getting tailored salt advice from healthcare professionals.

going over how certain health profiles, medications, and medical conditions should influence recommended sodium consumption.

4. Assessing Individual Health Goals: Examining how recommendations for salt intake may be influenced by specific health goals, such as controlling blood pressure or maintaining kidney health.

talking about how food decisions fit into certain senior health goals.

5. Modulating Sodium Consumption Based on Lifestyle Factors:

Understanding how lifestyle choices, such as total diet and physical activity, affect how much sodium is needed

talking about how modifying one's sodium consumption might support healthy, active senior living.

6. Balancing Taste Preferences with Health Goals:
Dealing with the difficulty of striking a balance between goals for reducing salt intake and flavor preferences

Investigating methods for sticking to the advised sodium intake while still eating a pleasurable and fulfilling diet

Factors Influencing Sodium Requirements in Aging Individuals

The complexity of dietary requirements changes as life's tapestry evolves, particularly with regard to sodium consumption for the elderly. This chapter explores the many variables that affect salt needs as people age gracefully and acknowledges that comprehensive knowledge is critical to making customized dietary decisions.

1. Physiological Changes with Aging: Examining how sodium metabolism is impacted by normal aging processes

talking about modifications to hydration levels, kidney function, and general physiology that affect salt requirements.

2. Kidney Function and Sodium Regulation: Examining how important the kidneys are in controlling the balance of sodium

talking about how renal function ages and how that affects salt excretion.

3. Medications and Health Conditions: Understanding how senior citizens' sodium balance is affected by their medications

going over how underlying medical issues, such as kidney disease or hypertension, might affect how much sodium is needed.

4. Individual Variability in Sensitivity: Recognizing that elderly people differ in their susceptibility to salt

talking about how certain seniors can be more vulnerable than others to the negative effects of consuming a lot of salt.

5. Physical Activity Levels: Examining how physical activity and salt needs are related

talking about how the activity levels of seniors who exercise regularly may affect how much sodium they require.

6. Dietary Patterns and Nutrient Intake: Understanding how dietary patterns and nutrient intake as a whole affect the amount of salt required

talking about how a balanced diet is essential for achieving dietary requirements and controlling salt intake.

7. Cultural and Lifestyle Influences: Discussing the ways in which lifestyle decisions and cultural preferences affect the amount of sodium consumed

talking about how dietary customs and tastes influence how much sodium an aging population needs.

8. Hydration Status: Stressing the link between salt balance and hydration

talking about how controlling salt levels in the body depends on preserving ideal hydration.

Consulting with Healthcare Professionals for Personalized Guidance

Healthcare professionals play a crucial role in achieving optimal health during one's golden years. This chapter emphasizes the value of getting individualized advice from medical professionals, giving seniors a road map to help them negotiate the complex world of salt intake based on their individual health profiles.

1. "Collaborative Health Approach"

stressing the importance of senior citizens and medical professionals working together to optimize health.

talking about how open communication promotes a mutual understanding of personal health objectives.

2. The significance: The significance of comprehensive health assessments carried out by healthcare providers is expounded upon in "Comprehensive Health Assessments.

going over how blood pressure, kidney function, and general health conditions affect the recommendations for sodium that are specific to each individual.

3. Medication Reviews and Interactions with Sodium:

acknowledging the possible influence of drugs on the equilibrium of sodium.

talking about the value of going over prescriptions with medical specialists to find any interactions and changes.

4. Customizing Sodium Recommendations: Examining how medical practitioners can alter sodium recommendations in accordance with patients' specific needs ·

talking about how to incorporate salt guidelines into general health management programs.

5. Traveling and Modifying Through Time:

stressing the need for continual monitoring and the dynamic nature of health.

talking about how medical professionals may be extremely helpful in modifying sodium recommendations when medical circumstances change.

6. Nutritional Counseling for Seniors: Acknowledging the role that nutritionists and licensed dietitians play in advising dietary decisions

going over the advantages of nutritional counseling for senior citizens, especially with regard to controlling their sodium intake.

7. Educating and Empowering Seniors: Stressing the need for healthcare providers to help seniors understand the significance of managing their sodium intake

talking about how people with more knowledge are better able to make lifestyle decisions that will improve their health.

8. Creating a Helpful Network: Promoting the creation of a senior-friendly healthcare network talking about the advantages of routine examinations and continuing contact with medical specialists in the pursuit of optimum health.

CHAPTER THREE

IDENTIFYING HIDDEN SODIUM IN DAILY FOODS

Uncovering Sneaky Sources of Salt in Common Foods

The secret to living a low-salt lifestyle is awareness. This chapter illuminates the sometimes disregarded and covert sources of salt woven throughout the fabric of everyday foods. Knowing these covert sources of sodium becomes an important tool for seniors starting the process of cutting back on their intake.

1. Foods treated and packed: determining the amount of salt that is hidden in foods that have been treated and packed

talking about how convenience foods affect the amount of sodium consumed overall and how to select low-sodium substitutes.

2. Conditions and Sauces: Dissecting the sodium that may be present in sauces and condiments

offering substitutes and home-cooked dishes that enhance flavor without sacrificing health.

3. Foods That Are Canted and Preserved: Examining How Much Sodium Is in Foods That Are Canted and Preserved

talking about how important it is to read labels and choose products with less or no added salt or sodium.

4. Delicious Bakeries and Deli Items: Finding the salt that is buried in these types of items

talking about how these seemingly harmless decisions can add a lot of sodium to one's daily intake.

5. Cheeses and Dairy Products: Analyzing the salt levels in different dairy products and cheeses

giving advice on how to choose options with less sodium and to make thoughtful decisions.

6. Restaurant and Takeout Meals: Drawing attention to the amount of salt found in these types of meals

talking about how to tell cooks about dietary restrictions and make educated decisions when dining out.

7. Instant and Ready-to-Eat Meals: Understanding the potential salt hazards associated with instant and ready-to-eat meals, notwithstanding their convenience

giving advice on how to make homemade substitutes or choose healthier ones.

8. Snack Foods and Salty Delights: Discovering the salt that lurks beneath the surface of salty delights and snack foods

offering suggestions for selecting snacks that satiate appetites without sacrificing health.

Reading Food Labels Effectively for Sodium Content

Understanding food labels becomes essential if one is trying to lead a low-salt diet. This chapter decodes nutrition label mysteries so that elders can accurately understand and analyze salt content and make well-informed choices.

1. Understanding Nutritional Facts Panels: Dissecting the Elements of Food Packaging Nutritional Facts Panels

talking about how serving sizes affect how much sodium is read.

2. Spotting Sodium Synonyms: Locating sodium under different names in ingredient lists

talking about the possible contributions of ingredients like sodium bicarbonate, sodium chloride, and monosodium glutamate (MSG) to total sodium intake.

3. Looking at Percent Daily Value (%DV): determining how much salt is recommended daily based on the amount on nutrition labels

talking about how determining a food item's sodium content can be made easier by using the %DV.

4. Comparing Products for Sodium Level: Compare the sodium level of similar products by using food labels.

going over how to select options with less sodium without sacrificing flavor or nutritional content.

5. Examining Ingredients for Hidden Sodium:

Examining ingredient lists closely for any unreported sodium sources

talking about the potential contributions of flavor enhancers, preservatives, and additives to total sodium levels.

6. Understanding Health Statements: Analyzing food packaging's statements about health related to sodium

talking about the meaning of phrases like "no added salt," "low sodium," and "reduced sodium."

7. Taking Portion Control into Account: Realizing how portion sizes affect the amount of salt consumed overall talking about the value of mindful eating and how consuming numerous portions can help meet daily sodium intake targets.

8. Using Mobile Apps and Online Resources: Examining how technology can be used to raise awareness about salt

talking about nutrient-dense smartphone apps and internet tools that make analyzing food labels simpler.

Cooking and Meal Preparation Tips for Minimizing Hidden Sodium

1. Embrace fresh ingredients: When constructing the base of your meals, choose fresh fruits, veggies, and meats. When it comes to sodium levels, fresh products typically have less than processed alternatives.

2. Spices and Herbs as Taste Enhancers: Try experimenting with different herbs and spices to give your food more flavor and complexity without using too much salt. Think about using herbs like cilantro, onion powder, rosemary, thyme, and garlic.

3. Citrus Zest and Juices: Incorporate natural brightness and tanginess into your recipes by using citrus zest and juices, such as orange, lemon, and lime, which will lessen the need for additional salt.

4. Homemade Stocks and Broths: You may manage the sodium content by making your own stocks and broths using fresh ingredients. This enhances the flavor of stews, sauces, and soups without having to use store-bought substitutes.

5. Reduce Processed Condiments: Keep in mind that salad dressings, ketchup, and soy sauce frequently include sodium that isn't readily apparent. To reduce the amount of salt, use low-sodium options or cook your own.

6. Rinse Canned Beans and Vegetables: Thoroughly rinse canned beans and vegetables under cold water before use to minimize salt content. Their salt level can be considerably reduced by taking this easy step.

7. Select Low-Sodium Substitutes: When available, choose low-sodium candies, broths, and other packaged foods. Examine product labels, do comparisons, and select items with the least amount of salt.

8. Limit the Use of Salt in Cooking: Lower the quantity of salt you use gradually when cooking. With time, your taste buds will adapt, and you'll be able to enjoy the items' authentic flavors.

9. Conscientious Meat Selection: Select lean, fresh meat, and poultry cuts because cured and processed meats typically contain a higher salt content. For more flavor, think about marinating meats with herbs and spices.

10. Discover Seasoning Blends Without Salt:

Try different herbs, spices, and dried aromatics to create your own unique twist, or try store-bought salt-free seasoning combinations.

11. Use Vinegars and Mustards: Add various vinegars (apple cider, balsamic) and mustards to improve flavor without using too much salt. These components can give your recipes more nuance and complexity.

12. Cooking Techniques to Preserve Flavor: Use cooking techniques like roasting, grilling, and sautéing that bring out the natural flavors in food. This enables you to achieve great outcomes with minimal salt.

13. Check the Labels for Low-Sodium Pasta and Bread: When buying bread and pasta goods, be sure to read the labels, as these may contain unreported sodium. Seek out products that are marked as sodium-free or low-sodium.

14. DIY Salad Dressings: Use vinegar, olive oil, spices, and herbs to make your own salad dressings. This gives you command over the components and removes needless sodium addition.

15. Teach Yourself About Sodium Content: Remain knowledgeable about the amount of sodium included in common ingredients. With this knowledge, you can plan and prepare meals with awareness and make informed decisions.

CHAPTER FOUR

CREATING A FLAVORFUL LOW SALT DIET PLAN

Exploring Alternative Seasonings and Herbs

Adding different herbs and seasonings to your cooking is a tasty way to expand your repertoire and give your food more depth while also lowering your dependency on sodium. By experimenting, you can change the way you season food and develop a palate of flavors that goes beyond just using salt.

1. Knowing the Effects of Salt Reduction: Acknowledge the advantages of cutting back on salt consumption for your health. Reducing sodium intake is associated with better blood pressure control and cardiovascular health, which is especially important for elderly people.

2. Natural Flavor Enhancers Using Herbs: Herbs are colorful, fragrant, and bursting with taste from nature. To improve the flavor of your food, add a range of fresh or dried herbs, such as cilantro, oregano, basil, rosemary, and thyme.

3. Try Different Spice Blends: Spice blends offer a well-balanced combination of tastes. In order to add complexity without adding more sodium, try international spice combinations like garam masala, za'atar, curry powder, and chili blends.

4. Juices and Zest of Citrus: The zesty flavor of citrus fruits, such as oranges, limes, and lemons, adds vibrancy to your food. To improve the taste of salads, marinades, and seafood dishes, grate in the zest or squeeze in some fresh juice.

5. Aromatics: Onions and Garlic: Whether they are roasted, minced, or fresh, garlic and onions add rich flavors to a variety of foods. Their flavorful attributes enhance both savory and sweet dishes, offering a gratifying substitute for salt.

6. Adding Flavor with Vinegars: Various vinegars, like red wine, apple cider, and balsamic, provide depth and acidity. Use them to improve flavor without using sodium in marinades, sauces, or dressings.

7. Umami-Enhancing Items: Add umami-rich items to your recipes, such as miso, tomatoes, and mushrooms. These components give off a savory flavor that is similar to the gratifying taste of salt but without the sodium.

8. Fresh and Dried Chilies: Use fresh or dried chilies to give your food a kick of spice and depth. Try several kinds, such as smoked paprika, Thai bird chilies, or jalapeños, to adjust the degree of heat to your taste.

9. Herbal Infusions: Steep fresh herbs, such as mint, basil, or thyme, in hot water to make herbal infusions. These infusions can be used as the foundation for drinks, soups, and sauces to add natural flavors to your food preparations.

10. Exploring Exotic Spices: To expand your flavor profile, use lesser-known spices like cardamom, coriander, and cumin. These spices add distinct flavors and fragrances to food that can elevate simple dishes to gourmet experiences.

11. In-house Sauces and Pesto: Make your own pesto by combining olive oil, pine nuts, garlic, and basil. Similarly, instead of using sodium-laden store-bought sauces, try making tasty sauces with roasted red peppers, sundried tomatoes, or roasted garlic.

12. Using Dried and Fresh Herbs in Salads: Add fresh herbs, such as cilantro, dill, or parsley, to salads to enhance their flavor. When added to homemade vinaigrettes, dried herbs provide a flavor boost without using too much salt.

13. "Culinary Oils Infused with Herbs: Try different herb-infused oils, such as grapeseed oil or olive oil infused with basil. They lessen the need for additional flavors while giving your food a mild herbal essence.

14. Combining Complementary Flavors: Recognize the subtleties of flavor combinations. To make recipes that are enjoyable and well-balanced, combine elements that go well together organically. Examples of this include combining acidic items with earthy spices or sweet fruits with savory herbs.

15. Learning About Flavor Profiles: Spend some time learning about the tastes of different spices and herbs. Knowing the various components that affect taste gives you the confidence to experiment and alter recipes to suit your tastes.

Cooking Techniques to Enhance Flavor Without Adding Salt

1. Searing for caramelization: Searing proteins, such as beef or tofu, in a hot skillet produces a golden-brown coating that can be used to heighten flavors without adding more salt.

2. Grilling for Smoky Notes: Foods that have been grilled acquire a noticeable smokiness. You can also try grilling fruits, veggies, and meats to add taste without adding salt.

3. Roasting for Depth: By concentrating the natural sugars in fruits, nuts, and vegetables, roasting them adds a pleasant richness without the need for additional salt.

4. Marinating for Infusion: Flavor layers are added to proteins by marinating them in blends of herbs, citrus, and aromatics. To improve flavor, let the ingredients steep in the marinade.

5. Poaching in Broths: This technique adds richness without using too much salt by poaching proteins in savory broths or stocks that are loaded with herbs and spices.

6. Using Aromatic Vegetables: To create a savory base and give your dishes depth and complexity without adding more salt, use aromatic vegetables like garlic, onions, and shallots.

7. Intensification through Slow Cooking: Slow cooking techniques enable flavors to gradually blend and amplify.

This method works especially well for making hearty soups, stews, and braised foods.

8. Basting for Moisture and Flavor: Without using salt, basting meats with liquids or oils flavored with herbs while they cook helps them retain moisture and add flavor.

9. "Sauteing with Aromatics": To give meals a deep and savory flavor, sauté aromatic herbs like rosemary, thyme, or sage while cooking veggies, proteins, or grains.

10. Deglazing for Flavorful Sauces: After cooking proteins, deglaze pans with liquids like wine, broth, or vinegar to extract concentrated flavors from the pan without adding salt.

11. Using Citrus Zest and Juice: Add zest and juice from citrus to dishes to make them pop. Without using salt, the acidity brings out the flavors and offers a cool contrast.

12. Fresh Herb Garnishes: Add a dash of fresh herbs, such as parsley, cilantro, or chives, to dishes to add a pop of flavor and visual appeal.

13. Infusing Oils with Herbs: Steep fresh herbs in oils, such as olive oil, to create herb-infused oils. Drizzle these oils over completed meals to bring out the herbal complexity even more.

14. Adding Layers of Flavor with Spices: Without using a salt shaker, add layers of flavor to your meals by layering in spices like paprika, coriander, and cumin.

15. Reducing and Concentrating Sauces: By reducing liquids and sauces, you can concentrate flavors and enhance flavor without adding more salt.

16. Adding umami-rich foods: Use umami-rich foods, such as miso, tomatoes, or mushrooms, to give food a savory, pleasing flavor without using a lot of sodium.

17. Using Nutritional Yeast: Nutritional yeast is a great way to enhance flavor without adding all the sodium of traditional cheese. It gives food a cheese-like flavor.

18. Toasting Nuts and Seeds: Toasting nuts and seeds adds a crunchy texture and boosts flavor in salads, side dishes, and even desserts by intensifying their nuttiness.

19. Blending Flavors in Compound Butters: Softened butter can be combined with citrus zest, herbs, or spices to make compound butters. Use these flavored butters to enhance the flavor and richness of a variety of recipes.

20. Try New Exotic Vinegars: In order to add acidity and complexity to your food without using more salt, try new vinegars like balsamic, sherry, or fruit-infused vinegars.

Sample Meal Plans Tailored for Seniors

Creating a well-balanced and flavorful meal plan for seniors involves incorporating nutrient-dense foods while considering individual dietary preferences and restrictions. Here's a sample four-week meal plan with accompanying recipes designed with seniors' health and enjoyment in mind. Please note that these meal plans are general in nature, and it's crucial to consider individual nutritional needs and consult with healthcare professionals for personalized guidance.

Day 1:

- **Breakfast:** Greek Yogurt Parfait with Fresh Berries and Almonds
- **Lunch:** Grilled Chicken Salad with Mixed Greens, Cherry Tomatoes, and Balsamic Vinaigrette
- **Dinner:** Baked Salmon with Lemon-Dill Sauce, Quinoa, and Steamed Broccoli

Day 2:

- **Breakfast**: Oatmeal with Sliced Banana and Walnuts
- **Lunch:** Turkey and Vegetable Wrap with Whole Grain Tortilla

- **Dinner:** Vegetable Stir-Fry with Tofu, Brown Rice, and Ginger-Soy Sauce

Day 3:

- **Breakfast:** Spinach and Feta Omelette with Whole Wheat Toast
- **Lunch:** Lentil Soup with a Side of Mixed Greens
- **Dinner:** Baked Chicken Breast with Sweet Potato Mash and Green Beans

Day 4:

- **Breakfast:** Whole Grain Pancakes with Fresh Berries and Maple Syrup
- **Lunch:** Quinoa Salad with Chickpeas, Cucumber, and Lemon-Tahini Dressing
- **Dinner:** Shrimp and Vegetable Skewers with Quinoa Pilaf

Day 5:

- **Breakfast:** Fruit Smoothie with Spinach, Banana, and Greek Yogurt
- **Lunch:** Caprese Salad with Tomato, Mozzarella, and Basil
- **Dinner:** Baked Cod with Herbed Couscous and Roasted Asparagus

Day 6:

- **Breakfast:** Cottage Cheese with Pineapple and Almond Slices
- **Lunch:** Chicken Caesar Salad Wrap with Whole Wheat Tortilla
- **Dinner:** Eggplant Parmesan with Whole Grain Pasta

Day 7:

- **Breakfast:** Whole Grain Toast with Avocado and Poached Egg
- **Lunch:** Quinoa and Black Bean Bowl with Avocado Salsa
- **Dinner:** Beef and Vegetable Stir-Fry with Brown Rice

Day 8:

- **Breakfast:** Banana Walnut Muffins with a Side of Yogurt
- **Lunch:** Turkey and Cranberry Sandwich on Whole Grain Bread
- **Dinner:** Grilled Vegetable and Chickpea Salad with Lemon-Tahini Dressing

Day 9:

- **Breakfast:** Blueberry-Almond Smoothie Bowl
- **Lunch:** Spinach and Feta Stuffed Chicken Breast with Roasted Brussels Sprouts
- **Dinner:** Baked Tilapia with Mango Salsa, Quinoa, and Steamed Broccoli

Day 10:

- **Breakfast:** Veggie Omelette with Whole Grain English Muffin
- **Lunch:** Greek Salad with Grilled Chicken and Tzatziki Dressing
- **Dinner:** Vegetarian Chili with Cornbread

Day 11:

- **Breakfast:** Overnight Chia Pudding with Mixed Berries
- **Lunch:** Turkey and Vegetable Stir-Fry with Brown Rice
- **Dinner:** Baked Zucchini Boats with Ground Turkey and Quinoa

Day 12:

- **Breakfast:** Whole Wheat Bagel with Smoked Salmon, Cream Cheese, and Capers

- **Lunch:** Lentil and Vegetable Curry with Basmati Rice
- **Dinner:** Lemon Herb Grilled Pork Chops with Sweet Potato Wedges

Day 13:

- **Breakfast:** Peanut Butter Banana Toast on Whole Grain Bread
- **Lunch:** Tuna Salad Lettuce Wraps with Tomato and Cucumber
- **Dinner:** Roasted Chicken Thighs with Mashed Cauliflower and Green Beans

Day 14:

- **Breakfast:** Apple Cinnamon Baked Oatmeal
- **Lunch:** Quinoa and Vegetable Stuffed Peppers
- **Dinner:** Spaghetti Squash with Marinara Sauce and Turkey Meatballs

Day 15:

- **Breakfast:** Mixed Berry Smoothie with Protein Powder
- **Lunch:** Chicken and Vegetable Kabobs with Quinoa Pilaf

- **Dinner:** Baked Cod with Tomato-Basil Relish, Brown Rice, and Steamed Asparagus

Day 16:

- **Breakfast:** Avocado and Tomato Breakfast Sandwich on Whole-Grain English Muffin
- **Lunch:** Chickpea Salad with Cucumber, Tomato, and Feta
- **Dinner:** Vegetable and Shrimp Stir-Fry with Cauliflower Rice

Day 17:

- **Breakfast:** Greek Yogurt Parfait with Granola and Sliced Peaches
- **Lunch:** Quinoa Salad with Roasted Vegetables and Feta Cheese
- **Dinner:** Baked Chicken Thighs with Herbed Sweet Potato Wedges and Green Beans

Day 18:

- **Breakfast:** Spinach and Mushroom Breakfast Burrito with Whole Wheat Tortilla
- **Lunch:** Turkey and Avocado Wrap with Spinach and Whole Grain Bread

- **Dinner:** Grilled Salmon with Lemon-Dill Marinade, Quinoa, and Steamed Broccoli

Day 19:

- **Breakfast:** Whole Grain Waffles with Fresh Strawberries and Whipped Cream
- **Lunch:** Lentil and Vegetable Soup with a Side of Mixed Greens
- **Dinner:** Stir-Fried Tofu with Vegetables and Brown Rice

Day 20:

- **Breakfast:** Cottage Cheese Pancakes with Blueberry Compote
- **Lunch:** Mediterranean Chickpea Salad with Cucumber, Tomato, and Olives
- **Dinner:** Roasted Vegetable Lasagne with a Side of Garlic Bread

Day 21:

- **Breakfast:** Berry and Almond Smoothie with Spinach
- **Lunch:** Chicken Caesar Salad with Whole Grain Croutons

- **Dinner:** Grilled Shrimp Skewers with Quinoa Pilaf and Asparagus

Day 22:

- **Breakfast:** Avocado Toast with Poached Egg and Cherry Tomatoes
- **Lunch:** Quinoa Bowl with Black Beans, Corn, Avocado, and Lime Vinaigrette
- **Dinner:** Baked Cod with Mediterranean Salsa, Brown Rice, and Roasted Brussels Sprouts

Day 23:

- **Breakfast:** Banana Walnut Muffins with a Side of Yogurt
- **Lunch:** Caprese Quinoa Salad with Balsamic Glaze
- **Dinner:** Vegetable and Chicken Stir-Fry with Ginger-Soy Sauce and Quinoa

Day 24:

- **Breakfast:** Whole Wheat Bagel with Cream Cheese, Smoked Salmon, and Capers
- **Lunch:** Turkey and Vegetable Stir-Fry with Brown Rice

- **Dinner:** Eggplant Parmesan with Whole Grain Pasta

Day 25:

- **Breakfast**: Blueberry-Almond Smoothie Bowl
- **Lunch:** Spinach and Feta Stuffed Chicken Breast with Roasted Brussels Sprouts
- **Dinner:** Baked Tilapia with Mango Salsa, Quinoa, and Steamed Broccoli

Day 26:

- **Breakfast:** Veggie Omelette with Whole Grain English Muffin
- **Lunch:** Greek Salad with Grilled Chicken and Tzatziki Dressing
- **Dinner:** Vegetarian Chili with Cornbread

Day 27:

- **Breakfast:** Overnight Chia Pudding with Mixed Berries
- **Lunch:** Turkey and Cranberry Sandwich on Whole Grain Bread
- **Dinner:** Grilled Vegetable and Chickpea Salad with Lemon-Tahini Dressing

Day 28:

- **Breakfast:** Whole Grain Pancakes with Fresh Berries and Maple Syrup

- **Lunch:** Quinoa Salad with Chickpeas, Cucumber, and Lemon-Tahini Dressing

- **Dinner:** Shrimp and Vegetable Skewers with Quinoa Pilaf

CHAPTER FIVE

PRACTICAL TIPS FOR DINING OUT ON A LOW SALT DIET

Navigating Restaurant Menus for Low Sodium Options

While dining out can be enjoyable, carefully reading restaurant menus is essential for seniors who are devoted to a low-sodium lifestyle. This chapter functions as a manual, providing doable tactics for making well-informed decisions when dining out and giving preference to lower-sodium selections.

1. Menu Exploration: Before placing an order, carefully go over the menu. Look for terms like "roasted," "steamed," or "grilled," as they typically denote less salty and healthier cooking techniques.

2. Dialogue with Waitstaff: Never be afraid to ask questions of the restaurant staff. Tell the servers that you prefer low-sodium foods, and inquire about any specific requests or sodium content information that they may supply.

3. Customizing Orders: A lot of eateries allow for dish customization. To reduce sodium intake, ask for adjustments like lowering or eliminating the salt used during preparation or requesting side dishes of sauces and dressings.

4. Selecting Fresh Starters: Choose starters that have had little processing and are fresh. Fresh fruit plates, vegetable-based appetizers, and salads with vinaigrette dressings are a good way to start a meal that is low in sodium.

5. Lean Protein Selections: Opt for lean protein sources like tofu, fish, or grilled chicken. Generally speaking, these options have less salt than highly processed or cured meats.

6. Sauces and Dressings on the Side: Ask for condiments, dressings, and sauces to be served side by side. This lowers the possibility of hidden salt in these flavor enhancers by letting you regulate how much you use.

7. Consider Your Sides Carefully: Choose your side dishes wisely. Instead of choosing sides like fries or highly seasoned rice that could be rich in salt, go for steamed vegetables, baked potatoes, or nutritious grains.

8. Discovering Diverse Culinaries: Investigate ethnic food cultures that are renowned for their use of diverse herbs and spices in their cooking. Middle Eastern,

Japanese, and Mediterranean cuisines frequently provide tasty options with less sodium.

9. Grilled and Roasted Options: Select foods that have been broiled, grilled, or roasted. These cooking techniques bring out the flavors in food naturally without using too much salt.

10. Watch Out for Hidden Sodium: Watch out for hidden salt sources, including marinades, soups, and broths. Find out how much salt is in these foods, or if you're not sure, think about avoiding them.

11. Share Huge amounts: Take into account splitting up big amounts with a dining partner. This encourages conscious eating and lets you enjoy a range of foods without going overboard with sodium.

12. Water Hydration: Choose water to stay hydrated rather than high-sodium drinks. In addition to promoting general health, water also helps the body's sodium levels stay balanced.

13. Reading Online Reviews: Use internet reviews to determine how salt-conscious a restaurant is. You can make better decisions if other diners can enlighten you on the sodium content of certain foods.

14. Being Ready with Substitutes: Make a list of the most popular low-sodium dining establishments in your neighborhood. In this manner, you can choose restaurants that suit your dietary requirements with confidence.

15. Rejoicing with Dessert Intentionally: If dessert is on the menu, choose something with less added sugar, sorbet, or fresh fruit. Generally speaking, these options have less sodium than highly processed treats.

Communicating Dietary Restrictions to Restaurant Staff

Seniors with dietary limitations, especially those on a low-sodium diet, must effectively communicate with restaurant workers. In addition to giving elders helpful advice on how to communicate their dietary preferences in a restaurant setting, this chapter emphasizes the value of aggressive and clear communication.

1. Be Clear and Specific: Clearly state what foods you are restricted to, including whether you must eat a low-sodium meal. It's important to communicate the value of reducing the amount of salt in your food in plain words.

2. Inform Early in the Dining Process: Let the restaurant know about any dietary restrictions as soon as you can, ideally when you make your reservation or arrive. This gives the kitchen crew enough time to create a specially ordered dish.

3. Ask Questions Regarding Preparation Techniques: Find out how food is seasoned, cooked, and prepared. Find out if the cook can comply with your request for little to no salt applied throughout the cooking procedure.

4. Request Nutritional Information: If available, ask for specifics on the amount of sodium or other nutrients in a particular menu item. Certain restaurants may have this information available on their website or may provide it upon request.

5. Use positive language: Present your dietary limitations favorably. Rather than stating, "I can't have salt," say, "I'm following a low-sodium diet for health reasons, and I appreciate your assistance in preparing a flavorful, low-sodium meal."

6. Emphasize Health Concerns: If at ease, briefly describe any ailments or health issues that call for a low-sodium diet. This can aid in the restaurant staff's comprehension of the significance of your dietary requirement.

7. Show Your Appreciation: Thank the establishment for making an effort to meet your dietary requirements. Both sides may cooperate and enjoy the meal more when there is a good and appreciative tone.

8. Talk About Substitutions: Find out if there are any alternatives to high-sodium items. For instance, find out if they can improve flavor without using salt by using herbs, spices, or other seasonings.

9. Give documented instructions: Provide a documented list of any dietary preferences or limits, if applicable. This can lower the possibility of misunderstandings by providing the kitchen workers with a visual reference.

10. Inform Through Apps or Reservation Platforms: When booking a reservation, inform the restaurant of any dietary restrictions using apps or reservation platforms. Users on certain platforms can leave notes or make unique requests for the eatery.

11. Ask the Chef's Opinion: If the chef is accessible, think about making an appointment to talk with them face-to-face. Chefs can offer advice on creating a personalized low-sodium meal and are frequently open to direct conversation.

12. If Required, Utilize Visual Aids: Consider illustrating dietary limits with straightforward diagrams or visual aids for better visual understanding. This can be very useful for communicating precise directions about preferred ingredient types.

13. Promote Open Dialogue: Promote candid conversations between you and the restaurant employees. In the event of doubts or inquiries, working together promotes a satisfying dining experience.

14. Give Feedback: Following the dinner, let the restaurant know how well the low-sodium preparation went. Positive comments highlight how crucial it is to accommodate a range of dietary requirements.

15. Plan Ahead for Special Occasions: Let people know in advance if you have dietary requirements if you're going to be dining out for a special event, like a birthday or anniversary. This enables the restaurant to set up everything required for a special dining experience.

Enjoying Social Gatherings While Maintaining a Low Salt Lifestyle

Social events offer chances for celebration and interaction, making them an essential component of life. Seniors who are dedicated to a low-salt lifestyle must strike a balance between following their dietary restrictions and having fun at social gatherings. This chapter provides seniors with helpful tips on how to attend social events to the fullest while limiting their sodium consumption.

1. Open Communication: Let the host or organizer know in advance what foods you prefer. This guarantees that low-sodium options are accessible and enables them to take your needs into account when creating the menu.

2. Bring a dish to share. Provide the party with a low-sodium dish. This not only ensures you have a satisfying and appetizing option to enjoy, but it also introduces others to scrumptious and healthful options.

3. Educate Friends and Family: Inform your friends and family about your low-salt way of living. They can support you and make thoughtful meal preparations and selections if they are informed about your dietary choices.

4. Plan Ahead: If at all feasible, find out the meal alternatives or menu prior to the event. It helps to know what to anticipate so that you may make plans and, if needed, have a small low-sodium meal in advance.

5. Hydrate Well: Drink plenty of water to stay hydrated when attending social events. In addition to promoting general health, enough hydration helps counteract the negative consequences of consuming more sodium.

6. "Savor Mindfully: Eat with awareness when in social situations. By taking your time and enjoying every bite, you may completely appreciate the flavors without going overboard with high-sodium foods.

7. Make an Informed Selection from the Buffet: When at a buffet, go over everything available before filling your plate. Pick a variety of low-sodium foods, like fresh produce, lean meats, and fruits.

8. "Personalize Your Plate Feel free to personalize your platter. Ask for adjustments to suit your low-sodium requirements, such as grilled foods or side sauces.

9. Seek Out Fresh Products: Give minimally processed and fresh products priority. Salads, fruit platters, and vegetable trays are examples of foods that are low in salt and offer a cool substitute.

10. Avoid Consuming Too Much Alcohol: Drink in moderation because some alcoholic beverages have a lot of salt in them. Select products with less salt and limit your consumption.

11. Create Flavorful Substitutes: Try out tasty substitutes for conventional high-sodium items. Use citrus, herbs, and spices, for instance, to improve flavor without using salt.

12. Host Your Own Gathering: Take charge of the menu by organizing get-togethers for yourself. This lets you share your favorite foods with others and make a spread that fits your low-sodium lifestyle.

13. Participate in Physical Activities: Strike a balance between socializing and exercising. Play social games or do mild exercise to improve your general health and lessen the effects of occasionally consuming more salt.

14. Exercise Portion Control: Pay attention to serving sizes. Eat less when enjoying social events, and pay attention to your body's signals of fullness.

15. Bring Low-Sodium Snacks: Pack your own low-sodium munchies to enjoy throughout the gathering. This guarantees that you have filling options without depending on party snacks that could be high in sodium.

16. Celebrate Non-Food Traditions: Reorient social events so that they are less about food-related activities. To add variety to the celebration, include non-food customs like storytelling, games, and arts and crafts.

17. Make Connections with Like-Minded People: Look for and establish connections with people who have similar dietary choices. It can be enjoyable and beneficial to share experiences and advice with like-minded people.

18. Retain a Positive Attitude: Approach social events with a constructive attitude. Accept the pleasure of mingling with others and place more emphasis on the relationships and experiences than the cuisine.

CHAPTER SIX

MANAGING HEALTH CONDITIONS WITH A LOW SALT DIET

Impact of Sodium Reduction on Hypertension and Cardiovascular Health

Seniors who want to put their health first must comprehend the connection between sodium consumption, hypertension, and cardiovascular health. The substantial effects of lowering sodium intake on controlling hypertension and enhancing general cardiovascular health are examined in this chapter.

1. "The Sodium Connection Between Hypertension: Examine the direct connection between elevated blood pressure and sodium intake. An excessive amount of sodium can cause fluid retention, which makes blood vessels work harder and raises blood pressure.

2. Reducing the Risk of Stroke: Talk about how cutting back on sodium intake can reduce the risk of stroke. Lowering sodium intake is essential for controlling blood pressure, which in turn lowers the risk of strokes and other cardiovascular events.

3. Heart Health Benefits: Consider the advantages of lowering salt intake for heart health. Reducing sodium intake lowers the risk of heart disease, heart attacks, and other cardiovascular problems by lessening the strain on the heart.

4. Managing Fluid Balance: Examine how lowering sodium helps the body's fluid balance to remain ideal. For seniors, this is especially important because imbalances can put stress on the heart and worsen cardiovascular problems.

5. Role in Kidney Function: Talk about the link between better kidney function and lowering sodium intake. Limiting sodium intake can help seniors' renal health, especially if they have age-related abnormalities in kidney function.

6. Collaboration with Medication: Emphasize how taking drugs for hypertension and reducing salt can work together. When seniors take medicine for hypertension, they can improve the efficacy of their treatment by also implementing a low-sodium diet.

7. Blood Pressure Regulation: Describe how lowering salt levels is essential for controlling blood pressure. Reducing sodium intake aids in better blood pressure regulation, which eases the burden on the cardiovascular system.

8. Adopting a Heart-Healthy Lifestyle: stress that cutting back on salt is an essential part of living a heart-healthy lifestyle in general. This entails controlling stress levels, keeping a healthy weight, and engaging in regular physical activity.

9. Personalized Methods: Acknowledge that every person's reaction to sodium consumption may be different. Customized strategies for reducing salt intake are crucial since certain people, particularly the elderly, may be more sensitive to the mineral.

10. Educational Initiatives: Talk about the significance of senior citizen education regarding the effects of sodium on cardiovascular health. Giving seniors access to resources and information enables them to make educated decisions about their nutrition and way of life.

11. Seniors' Long-Term Advantages: Emphasize the long-term advantages of lowering salt intake for senior citizens. Living a low-sodium lifestyle can help maintain cardiovascular health for longer, which can support an improved quality of life as we age.

12. Encouraging Elders to Make Informed Decisions: Encourage elders to actively participate in their cardiovascular health by making knowledgeable dietary decisions. This entails reading food labels, identifying sodium's hidden sources, and choosing healthier foods.

13. Working Together with Healthcare Professionals: Stress the value of working together with healthcare professionals. Seniors who visit their doctors on a regular basis can get tailored advice and guidance on controlling their hypertension and cutting back on sodium consumption.

14. Supporting Community Promotion: Talk about how important it is for the community to promote heart-healthy behaviors. Seniors can commit to cardiovascular health as a group by participating in community programs, support groups, or educational activities.

15. Sodium Intake Monitoring: Give elders helpful advice on how to keep an eye on and cut back on their sodium intake. This includes reading food labels, selecting whole, fresh foods, and exercising caution when using cooking techniques that could release unintentional sodium sources.

Dietary Approaches for Seniors with Kidney Concerns

Careful consideration of food choices is necessary for seniors with kidney issues to maintain overall health and kidney health. This chapter explores realistic dietary strategies designed for older adults with kidney problems, offering advice on nutritional intake, fluid consumption, and lifestyle modifications.

1. Knowing How the Kidney Works: Start by describing how the kidneys remove waste products and extra fluid from the blood. Dietary advice is based on a thorough understanding of renal function.

2. Importance of Low Sodium Intake: Stress the need to stick to a low-sodium diet for people who have kidney issues. Lowering sodium consumption eases the burden on the kidneys and helps maintain fluid balance.

3. Managing Fluid Intake: Talk about how crucial it is to keep an eye on fluid intake. It may be necessary for seniors who have kidney issues to control how much fluid they consume in order to avoid overtaxing their kidneys. Customize recommendations in accordance with medical advice and each person's needs.

4. Balancing Protein Consumption: Examine the careful equilibrium of protein consumption. Seniors who are concerned about their kidneys may need to modify their protein intake; choose high-quality sources and limit their intake overall to lessen the strain on their kidneys.

5. Reduced Phosphorus Consumption: Talk about how phosphorus affects renal function. Restricting phosphorus-rich diets can help seniors with kidney problems avoid imbalances that can exacerbate heart and bone problems.

6. Selecting Kidney-Friendly Proteins: Provide an inventory of protein sources that are suitable for kidneys. Lean meat consumption is supported by including plant-based proteins like beans and tofu, which don't put undue strain on the kidneys.

7. Keeping an Eye on Potassium Levels: Talk about how important it is to keep an eye on potassium levels in the diet. Seniors who have kidney issues might need to control how much potassium they eat to avoid problems from high amounts.

8. Maximizing Calcium Intake: Consider how calcium affects renal function. Urge elderly people to maximize their calcium intake from low-phosphorus sources in order to support bone health without aggravating renal issues.

9. Putting a Focus on Fruits and Vegetables: Promote the eating of fruits and vegetables. Seniors can reap the benefits of these foods' minerals and antioxidants, which boost general health, while keeping an eye on potassium levels.

10. Restricting Foods Rich in Phosphorus: Draw attention to the fact that processed and quick meals should be avoided since they frequently contain additives that raise phosphorus levels. Urge senior citizens to limit their intake of phosphorus by selecting whole, unprocessed foods.

11. Cooking Techniques for Kidney Health: Talk about cooking techniques that are good for the kidneys. Generally speaking, it is better to grill, roast, or boil food because these methods help preserve nutrients and reduce the need for additional salt and spice.

12. Personalized Meal Scheduling: Emphasize the value of customized meal planning. Based on their overall health, the severity of their kidney problems, and other personal considerations, each person may require a different diet.

13. Journaling and Nutrient Monitoring: Advocate for journaling and nutrient monitoring. Informed decisions on dietary adjustments can be made by seniors and their healthcare providers by keeping note of daily food intake, fluid consumption, and pertinent lab findings.

14. Cooperating with a dietician: Stress the importance of collaborating with a certified dietician. A dietitian can help elders achieve maximum renal health via nutrition, offer individualized assistance, and customize dietary recommendations to meet specific needs.

15. Including Lifestyle Modifications: Look at lifestyle modifications outside of nutrition. Maintaining a healthy weight, controlling stress, and getting enough sleep all improve general wellbeing and kidney health.

Collaborating with Healthcare Providers for Optimal Health Management

Seniors who want to take an active role in managing their health must effectively collaborate with healthcare practitioners. This chapter delves into the importance of forming solid relationships with medical professionals and provides guidance on communication, routine check-ups, and the role of a multidisciplinary approach in the best possible management of health.

1. Establishing Open Communication: Stress the value of candid communication between patients and healthcare professionals. Seniors should be encouraged to openly discuss any health issues, lifestyle modifications, or difficulties they may be experiencing.

2. Regular Health Check-ups: Emphasize the importance of routine health examinations. Regular visits let medical professionals keep an eye on patients' health, identify possible problems early, and modify treatment programs as necessary.

3. Understanding Medication Management: Talk about how important it is to comprehend and follow medication management. Seniors need to know the goals of the drugs they are prescribed, as well as any possible negative effects. Optimal pharmacological therapy is ensured by routinely discussing drugs with healthcare experts.

4. Collaboration with Experts: Examine the advantages of working with experts. Seniors may find it helpful to meet with experts like dietitians, physical therapists, or mental health specialists to address particular parts of their well-being, depending on their unique health needs.

5. Examining Diagnostic Tests and Lab Results: Motivate elders to participate in active conversations regarding their diagnostic tests and lab results. By comprehending these findings, individuals can take an active role in managing their health and make well-informed decisions regarding lifestyle modifications.

6. Disclosure of Lifestyle Modifications: Emphasize the value of informing medical professionals of any changes in lifestyle. Notifying healthcare providers about new workout regimens, nutritional alterations, or daily routine adjustments allows them to offer customized advice and assistance.

7. Setting Realistic Health Goals: Assist elders in working with their healthcare providers to establish reasonable health goals. Setting attainable goals encourages motivation and a sense of success along the health management path.

8. Managing chronic difficulties: Talk about practical methods for dealing with long-term medical difficulties. Comprehensive management regimens, which may involve medication, lifestyle modifications, and continuous monitoring, are beneficial for seniors with persistent health difficulties.

9. Preventive Healthcare Measures: Stress the significance of taking preventive action in healthcare. Early detection and prevention of health problems can be greatly aided by routine tests, vaccines, and lifestyle modifications.

10. Building a Health Information Binder: Provide advice on how to construct a health information binder. A thorough medical history, current prescriptions, recent lab results, and a list of queries or concerns for future doctor's appointments can all be found in this binder.

11. Promoting Personalized Care: Motivate elderly individuals to promote customized care. Seniors should actively communicate their preferences and concerns to receive care that is in line with their goals and values, as each person's health needs are unique.

12. Ask About Support Services: Ask about the support services that are offered. Seniors who need additional services to supplement their health management plan, such as support groups or community resources, might be connected by healthcare providers.

13. "Taking Part in Shared Decision-Making: Encourage seniors and healthcare professionals to collaborate on decisions. Seniors ought to have the confidence to actively engage in decisions on their lifestyle, course of treatment, and general health.

14. Understanding Insurance Coverage: Inform senior citizens about the coverage provided by their insurance. Understanding the scope of coverage for different healthcare treatments guarantees access to essential care and helps avoid unexpected shocks.

15.Regular Updates on Health Education: Promote frequent updates on health education. Seniors who keep up to date on pertinent health issues are better able to make informed decisions about their health and actively participate in discussions with healthcare professionals.

CHAPTER SEVEN

OVERCOMING CHALLENGES AND RESISTANCE TO A LOW SALT LIFESTYLE

Addressing Common Concerns and Misconceptions

Seniors who want to make educated decisions about their health must be able to navigate health-related issues and dispel myths. This chapter dispels common worries and myths, offering clarification on a range of health-related issues and encouraging a more precise comprehension.

1. The myth that all fats are unhealthy: Describe the differences between fats that are beneficial and unhealthy. Stress how crucial it is to include foods high in unsaturated fats, including nuts and avocados, in a balanced diet.

2. Apprehension:

Exercise Is Only Suitable for the Young: Dispel the misconception that exercise is solely appropriate for the young. Emphasize the advantages of consistent physical activity for senior citizens, such as better mood, increased mobility, and improved cardiovascular health.

3. Myth: Mental Sharpness Declines with Age: Dispel the myth that aging causes a natural reduction in mental acuity. Emphasize the value of lifelong learning, social interaction, and mental exercise in preserving cognitive function.

4. Apprehension:

 Losing Weight Is Always Beneficial: Dispel the myth that losing weight automatically translates into better health. Emphasize the value of managing weight in a balanced manner, concentrating on general health rather than just the number on the scale.

5. Myth: A Healthy Diet Can Be Replaced by Supplements Make it clear that although supplements can be a good addition to a balanced diet, they cannot take the place of whole meals in terms of nutrients. Seniors should be urged to prioritize eating a varied, nutrient-rich diet.

6. Apprehension: Sleep Requirements Drop with Age: Reject the idea that sleep requirements drop with age. Stress the significance of regular and adequate sleep for seniors' general health, emotional stability, and cognitive function.

7. Myth: Strength Training Isn't Good for Seniors Dispel the myth that elderly people should stay away from strength training because they are more likely to get hurt. Draw attention to the advantages of strength exercise for preserving bone density, muscle mass, and functional independence.

8. Apprehension:

It's Too Late to Give Up Smoking: Disprove the notion that it's too late to stop smoking as you age. Emphasize the short- and long-term health advantages of quitting smoking, such as enhanced respiratory health and a lower risk of cardiovascular disease.

9. Myth: Vaccinations Are Not Needed by Older Adults Make clear the significance of immunizations for senior citizens. Dispel the misconception that vaccinations are just for kids by highlighting how they can protect the elderly from life-threatening diseases and their consequences.

10. Apprehension:

Persistent Pain Is Unavoidable as One Ages Disprove the notion that aging and chronic pain are synonymous. Emphasize the need for preserving joint health, continuing an active lifestyle, and obtaining the right medical attention in order to manage and prevent chronic pain.

11. Myth: Seniors Shouldn't Bother with Healthy Eating: Dispel the illusion that older citizens don't need to follow a healthy diet. Stress the importance of diet in maintaining energy levels, preventing chronic diseases, and promoting general health.

12. Apprehension: Isolation Is Unavoidable in Old Age: Dispel the fallacy that loneliness is an inherent aspect of aging. Urge elderly people to take an active part in social events that will strengthen their bonds with friends, family, and the community.

13. Myth: Alzheimer's Disease Is Always Associated with Memory Loss: Make it clear that forgetfulness sometimes is not a sign of dementia. Inform them that memory alterations are a natural part of aging and stress the need to consult a doctor if memory problems become persistent or worrisome.

14. Apprehension:

Seniors Must Not Take Up New Interests: Disprove the notion that elderly people shouldn't take up new interests or acquire new abilities. Stress the happiness that can arise from discovering new hobbies as well as the mental and emotional advantages of lifelong learning.

15. Myth: Experiencing Pain During Exercise: Dispel the myth that experiencing pain is a typical aspect of exercising. Seniors should be urged to differentiate between pain that comes with exercise and pain that could cause an injury, with an emphasis on the necessity of altering activities as necessary.

Strategies for Encouraging Family and Friends' Support

Establishing a network of family and friends who can provide support is crucial for seniors who want to continue living a healthy lifestyle. This chapter looks at practical methods for enticing and cultivating family support, which improves well-being by promoting a good atmosphere.

1. Open and Honest Communication: Stress the value of having honest and open communication with loved ones. Clearly state your worries and goals regarding your health, as well as the importance of their support in establishing and sustaining a healthy lifestyle.

2. Educate on Health Goals: Spend some time informing friends and family about particular health objectives. Whether it's maintaining an active lifestyle, avoiding salt, or handling stress, giving explanations for these decisions improves understanding and support.

3. Share Successes and Milestones: Congratulate loved ones on accomplishments and significant anniversaries. Whatever the size of the accomplishment, celebrating it together creates a sense of group achievement and highlights the beneficial effects of their support.

4. Involve Them in Activities: Involve friends and family in activities that pertain to their health. Whether it's preparing a nutritious meal together, taking walks, or engaging in group exercise programs, shared experiences fortify relationships and foster a nurturing atmosphere.

5. Request Accompanying Visits: Request their presence when attending medical visits. A loved one's presence can boost collaborative health talks, improve comprehension of medical information, and offer emotional support.

6. Host health-focused gatherings: arrange events that are health-focused. Organize gatherings that are focused on wholesome food, exercise, or wellness pursuits to foster an atmosphere that inevitably encourages making health-conscious decisions.

7. Provide Information on Healthy Practices: Disseminate details regarding the advantages of healthy practices. Giving friends and family the information, they need empowers them to make decisions that promote a healthy and supportive environment.

8. Express Particular Support Needs: Clearly state the particular ways in which they can provide assistance. Determining support needs enables loved ones to contribute more skillfully, whether it's helping with meal preparation, participating in fitness regimens, or offering encouragement.

9. Formula for Wellness Support Group Creation: Form a group for wellness support. Encourage your loved ones to join you in your dedication to good health by fostering a community where advice, encouragement, and experiences are freely exchanged.

10. Sponsor Healthy Activities: Promote cooperative healthy activities. Make recommendations for activities that support health objectives, including going on walks with a group, gardening, or attending wellness classes together.

11. Provide Resources and Literature: Provide enlightening literature and resources. To start a dialogue and foster a shared interest in leading healthier lives, share books, documentaries, or articles about health and wellbeing.

12. Exemplify healthy behaviors: Set a good example. Set a good example for others by modeling healthy practices on a regular basis. This will encourage others to make similar lifestyle choices.

13. Thank Them for Their Support: Thank them and appreciate their assistance. Expressing gratitude on a regular basis helps to fortify the relationship between you and your support system and reaffirms the significance of their contribution to your health journey.

14. Be Open to Their Feedback: Remain receptive to helpful criticism. In order to create a two-way communication channel that improves understanding between people, encourage family and friends to express their ideas and worries.

15. Celebrate Together: Honor group accomplishments. Reaching exercise goals, establishing new healthy routines, or hitting health milestones all enhance the sense of accomplishment that comes from celebrating as a group.

Motivational Techniques for Maintaining Long-Term Dietary Changes

Long-term dietary adjustments might be difficult to maintain, but seniors can stick to their health goals with the correct incentive techniques. This chapter looks at practical ways to encourage and support seniors as they make the switch to healthy eating habits.

1. Set achievable and reasonable goals: Help elders establish dietary objectives that are both attainable and reasonable. Divide more ambitious goals into more doable chunks, acknowledging and appreciating each small victory as you go.

2. Create a Vision Board: Encourage the making of a vision board that illustrates your health objectives. Incorporate pictures, sayings, and affirmations that will act as a continual reminder of the advantages of making dietary adjustments.

3. Create a Support Network: Stress the value of having a robust support network. Having people who support and hold you accountable, whether they be family, friends, or a health coach, may greatly increase motivation.

4. Eating with Mindfulness: Explain the idea of mindful eating. To help elders feel more connected to the food they eat, encourage them to savor every bite, pay attention to indications of hunger and fullness, and use all of their senses when dining.

5. Celebrate Small Wins: Honor modest accomplishments. Celebrate and acknowledge each successful dietary decision to help spread the message that any accomplishment, no matter how tiny, is a step in the right direction.

6. Discover New Cuisines and Recipes: Explore new cuisines and recipes to keep things interesting. Adding diversity to the diet keeps things interesting and injects some excitement into the process of choosing better foods.

7. Create a Routine: Assist elderly people in creating a routine. Long-term adherence to dietary modifications is facilitated by a sense of structure that is created by maintaining consistency in meal planning, preparation, and eating times.

8. Keep a Food Journal: Provide advice on maintaining a food diary. Daily meal and snack logs reveal eating patterns, point out possible areas for development, and provide concrete documentation of advancements.

9. Reward Yourself: Establish a system of prizes. Make a list of non-food incentives for reaching particular nutritional benchmarks to provide yourself with positive reinforcement to make better decisions.

10. Remain Educated on Health Advantages: Continue to educate people on the advantages of dietary modifications for their health. Knowing how these adjustments enhance general well-being can be a strong incentive.

11. Take Part in Regular Physical Activity: Stress the link between physical activity and diet. A comprehensive approach to health and well-being can be promoted by regular exercise in addition to dietary modifications.

12. Visualize Long-Term Health: Motivate elders to see how their food choices will affect their long-term health. Contemplating a brighter, healthier future might be a great way to stay motivated when things get hard.

13. Join Clubs or Cooking Classes: Encourage participation in clubs or cooking classes. Acquiring new culinary skills and exchanging tales with individuals undergoing comparable circumstances can provide motivation and a feeling of unity.

14. Practice Positive Affirmations: Include affirmations in your everyday activities. Remind seniors of their nutritional objectives by saying them out loud. This will help them feel empowered and have a good outlook.

15. Seek Professional Guidance: Stress how crucial it is to get professional advice. Dietitians, nutritionists, and other medical professionals can provide individualized guidance, handle issues, and offer continuing support for sticking to dietary modifications.

CHAPTER EIGHT

MONITORING SODIUM INTAKE AND TRACKING PROGRESS

Establishing a System for Tracking Daily Sodium Consumption

One of the most important parts of maintaining a low-salt lifestyle is monitoring your daily sodium intake. This chapter offers advice on how to set up a workable system for seniors to track and control the amount of salt they consume, raising awareness and encouraging them to stick to a better diet.

1. Keep a Food Journal: Seniors should be urged to keep a food journal. Keep track of all the meals, snacks, and drinks you have during the day, along with any specifics like portion sizes and cooking techniques.

2. Utilize Mobile Apps: Introduce smartphone apps made to monitor salt consumption. Numerous apps enable users to record their daily meals, giving them fast access to salt content information and making monitoring simple.

3. Read Food Labels: Stress how important it is to read product labels. Teach elderly people how to read product labels for salt levels and to pay attention to serving sizes so they may make wise decisions when they go grocery shopping.

4. Make a spreadsheet to manage sodium: Assist seniors with making a customized spreadsheet to manage sodium. They can enter their daily salt intake into this straightforward template, which will make it easier to see patterns and pinpoint areas that need work.

5. Color-Coding System: Put in place a system of color coding. To provide a quick visual reference for daily consumption, assign different colors to different amounts of sodium concentration and use these colors to highlight entries in the food journal or spreadsheet.

6. Set Daily Sodium Goals: Establish daily sodium objectives in collaboration with elders. Establish reasonable goals based on each person's unique health needs in collaboration, and monitor your progress regularly.

7. Use a Sodium Calculator: Showcase sodium calculators available online. These technologies provide extra insights for efficient tracking by estimating salt consumption based on the kinds and quantities of meals consumed.

8. Review Progress Often: Plan frequent evaluations of sodium consumption. These evaluations, which might be weekly or monthly, offer a chance to evaluate development, recognize successes, and pinpoint areas that might require improvement.

9. Incorporate Visual Aids: Make charts or graphs to illustrate data on salt intake visually. Seniors who are visualizing trends over time may find it inspiring and easier to stay goal-focused.

10. Work with a dietician: Promote partnership with a dietician. A specialist can offer seniors continuous guidance in controlling their sodium intake as well as help them understand the tracking data they have collected.

11. Distribute Tracking Methods in Support Groups: If appropriate, join or start a support group. Building a sense of community and encouraging one another is facilitated by exchanging tracking strategies and experiences with those traveling a similar path.

12. Utilize a Kitchen Scale: Suggested usage is a kitchen scale. When making homemade meals or following recipes, seniors can more precisely determine the sodium level of the items by weighing them before cooking.

13. Pre-Plan Meals and Snacks: Promote organizing meals and snacks in advance. Anticipating ahead enables elderly individuals to make deliberate judgments, regulate their salt consumption, and steer clear of rash choices that could lead to excessive consumption.

14. Incorporate Takeout and Restaurant Information: Encourage elders to incorporate takeout and restaurant information into their tracking. When elders are dining out, a lot of eateries include nutritional information to help them make educated decisions.

15. Regularly Update Knowledge: Emphasize how important it is to keep up with the sodium content of different foods. Updating knowledge on a regular basis guarantees that elders can make educated dietary selections and are aware of hidden sources of salt.

Recognizing and Celebrating Milestones in Salt Reduction

Rewarding yourself for reaching new goals is essential to staying motivated and forming healthy habits. In order to give seniors a sense of accomplishment and strengthen their resolve to lead low-sodium lifestyles, this chapter examines practical methods for identifying and celebrating their successes in reducing their intake of salt.

1. Establish clear milestones: collaborate with seniors to set attainable and unambiguous benchmarks. These benchmarks could be completing a predetermined number of days within the suggested salt intake, navigating a social gathering with low-sodium options with ease, or cooking at home on a regular basis.

2. Make a Milestone Schedule: Make a milestone schedule. Putting noteworthy accomplishments on a calendar helps as a continuous reminder of the constructive actions taken toward a lower salt intake and offers a visual depiction of development.

3. Achievement Reward System: Establish a system of rewards for accomplishing goals. Give distinct prizes— like a soothing spa day, a beloved book, or a leisurely outdoor activity—for varying degrees of success.

4. Host a Celebration Meal: Organize a get-together or celebration meal. To celebrate reaching a milestone, make a special low-sodium meal and invite friends and family to join you in the celebration.

5. Write Personal Success Tales: Seniors should be urged to write up their individual success tales. Sharing their journey, whether through journaling, blogging, or making a video diary, can encourage others and reaffirm the beneficial effects of their work.

6. Share Achievements in Support Groups: Talk about your accomplishments with other members of your support group. Celebrating together creates a good atmosphere for continued success by fostering a sense of community and mutual support.

7. Build an acknowledgment board: Make a board for acknowledgment at home. Showcase accolades, encouraging words, or symbols that stand for accomplished goals to provide a concrete and visible reminder of accomplishment.

8. Organize a Physical Activity Challenge: Arrange a challenge including physical activity. Connect fitness goals with milestones, such as reaching a step count target, attempting a new workout, or taking part in a group exercise session.

9. Acknowledgment of Consistent Effort: Stress the significance of perseverance. Major achievements are important, but recognizing the everyday effort to consume less salt emphasizes the need for persistent commitment.

10. Take Part in a Culinary Journey: Go on a culinary journey. Celebrate your accomplishments by experimenting with new low-sodium dishes or inventive ways to flavor food without adding too much salt.

11. Build a Customized Certificate: Create customized certificates. Make success certificates for particular benchmarks to give the acknowledgment procedure more formality and weight.

12. Host a Virtual Celebration: If attending in-person events is difficult, consider hosting a virtual celebration. Use video conversations to stay in touch with loved ones and exchange accomplishments, tales, and well wishes.

13. Take Part in Gratitude and Reflection: Promote appreciation and introspection. Give yourself time to think back on the experience, be thankful for the help you've gotten, and acknowledge the personal development that comes with adopting a low-sodium diet.

14. Attend educational seminars or workshops: Go to seminars or workshops that are educational. Celebrate your accomplishments by learning more about wellness, nutrition, and health and by highlighting the link between continued learning and long-term success.

15. Incorporate Symbolic Representations: Include accomplishment symbols in your work. Having a physical representation of achievement, whether in the form of tokens, badges, or customized artwork, provides a constant reminder of advancement.

Adjusting the Diet Plan as Needed Based on Individual Responses

Long-term success in maintaining a low-sodium lifestyle requires tailoring the diet plan to each person's unique response. This chapter looks at methods that help older adults evaluate how they react to dietary changes and modify in a way that best suits their individual requirements and preferences.

1. Maintain a Symptom Journal: Suggest to elders that they maintain a symptom journal. Keeping track of the items they eat or the amount of sodium they consume might help shed light on each person's unique reaction.

2. Regularly assess energy levels: stress the significance of doing an energy level assessment on a frequent basis. Variations in tiredness, sluggishness, or alertness may be signs of how effectively the present food plan is promoting general health.

3. Check blood pressure: Promote routinely taking your blood pressure. In order to monitor blood pressure levels and determine whether dietary modifications are successfully assisting in blood pressure management, seniors can collaborate with medical specialists in this regard.

4. Assisting seniors: Assist seniors in identifying any indications of fluid retention by using the "Check for Fluid Retention" method. Ankle or other area swelling may indicate that dietary changes to minimize sodium intake are necessary to preserve the ideal fluid balance.

5. Evaluate Digestive Health: Emphasize how crucial it is to assess digestive health. Seniors should keep an eye on how dietary modifications impact their digestion, taking note of any discomfort, bloating, or anomalies that might call for alterations.

6. Evaluating Emotional Well-Being: Take emotional well-being into account. Modifications in diet can have an effect on emotional health and mood. Seniors should evaluate the effects of their food plan on their emotional and mental well-being.

7. Seek Advice from a Registered Dietician: Promote routine meetings with a registered dietician. These experts are able to offer tailored advice, assess each person's reaction to dietary modifications, and make educated modifications as necessary.

8. Incorporate flexibility into the plan: Make sure the diet plan is flexible. Acknowledge that every person will react differently and that a flexible strategy allows for modifications without sacrificing overall health objectives.

9. Try other flavors and seasonings: Offer trying other flavors and seasonings. It is possible to significantly reduce sodium intake while still enjoying delicious food by modifying the seasoning of meals.

10. Take Individual Sensitivities into Account: Take individual sensitivities into account. Certain foods may cause reactions in certain seniors due to allergies or unique sensitivities. Make appropriate adjustments to the diet plan to account for these variables.

11. Explore Other Low-Sodium Choices: Promote the investigation of other low-sodium choices. Seniors can find new ingredients and foods that offer variety and nutritional advantages while meeting their dietary goals.

12. Continually Examine Food Labels: Emphasize the value of reading food labels on a regular basis. Manufacturers may alter their formulations, so it's important for seniors to study labels carefully to make educated decisions and spot possible hidden salt sources.

13. Seek Professional Guidance for Changes: Suggest to elders that when making major changes, they should consult a professional. Consulting with healthcare providers before making any significant dietary plan changes, such as removing particular food groups, provides safe and well-informed choices.

14. Pay Attention to Your Body's Signals: Urge elderly people to pay attention to their bodies' cues. Understanding your hunger, fullness, and desires can help you make better nutritional decisions.

15. Remind seniors to stay informed about their own health goals: Encourage seniors to keep themselves updated on their own health goals. It's important to periodically review and evaluate these objectives to make sure the food plan is in line with overall well-being goals.

CHAPTER NINE

INTEGRATING PHYSICAL ACTIVITY AND LIFESTYLE CHOICES

Exploring the Connection Between Exercise and Sodium Balance

Seniors who want to maintain a healthy and balanced lifestyle must comprehend the complex relationship between activity and salt balance. This chapter examines how exercise affects sodium levels and offers suggestions for seniors on how to maximize their physical activity levels to maintain overall sodium balance.

1. Function of fluid control during exercise: Sweating involves the loss of both water and salt and is the body's natural cooling function. Seniors who engage in physical exercise should be careful to drink enough water.

2. Electrolyte Balance and Sodium Loss: Describe how sodium loss and electrolyte balance are related to one another when exercising. Sweating causes the loss of vital electrolytes, such as sodium, in addition to depleting water. It's essential to keep this equilibrium for general wellness.

3. Importance of Pre-activity Hydration: Stress the significance of hydrating before an activity session. In order to avoid the danger of dehydration during exercise and to ensure sodium balance, seniors should begin their physical activity properly hydrated.

4. Rehydration Strategies Post-Exercise: Talk about rehydration techniques after working out. Seniors should rehydrate after physical exertion in order to maintain balance and aid in healing. This includes salt and other electrolytes.

5. Identifying hyponatremia indicators: Provide instruction on identifying hyponatremia indicators. Although dehydration is a worry, imbalances can result from overhydration without enough sodium intake. Seniors need to be mindful of symptoms like headaches, nausea, and disorientation.

6. Hydration Suggestions for Various Activities: Adapt hydration suggestions to various activities. Depending on the length and intensity of the exercise, different amounts of liquid and sodium may be required. Seniors should modify their approach to hydration appropriately.

7. Building Balanced Meals Around Exercise: Motivate elders to build a healthy meal plan around their exercise regimen. Maintaining a balanced salt intake and a variety of carbs, proteins, and healthy fats when exercising helps to maintain energy levels.

8. Selecting Electrolyte-Rich Foods: Stress the significance of selecting foods high in electrolytes. When exercising, consuming foods high in potassium, like oranges and bananas, together with foods high in sodium, can improve the electrolyte balance overall.

9. Individual Differences in Sodium Requirements: Recognize that everyone has different sodium requirements. Seniors may require various amounts of sodium, depending on their age, health, and rate of perspiration during exercise. It's important to adjust sodium consumption.

10. Water Monitoring in Hot Weather: Stress the importance of increased water monitoring in hot weather. Sweating more frequently in hot weather can result in more salt loss. Seniors should modify their sodium and hydration consumption appropriately.

11. Avoiding Excessive Sodium Intake: Take care not to consume too much sodium. Even though sodium is necessary, seniors—especially those with certain medical conditions—should find a balance and refrain from overdoing themselves on salt.

12. Consulting healthcare specialists for assistance: Encourage seniors to seek individualized assistance from healthcare specialists. Individualized recommendations for salt intake during exercise may be beneficial for those with certain health issues or diseases.

13. Timing of Sodium Intake: Talk about when to take sodium. Seniors who engage in regular physical activity can maintain electrolyte balance by deliberately incorporating foods high in sodium into their pre- and post-exercise meals.

14. Taking Medication Interactions into Account: Talk about possible drug interactions. Seniors should be aware of how certain drugs may interfere with salt balance in order to make educated decisions about their diet and level of exercise.

15. Monitoring Individual Responses: Stress the significance of keeping an eye on each person's answer. Seniors should monitor how their bodies react to various salt and hydration tactics while exercising and make any necessary adjustments depending on their individual experiences.

Incorporating Senior-Friendly Physical Activities

For elders to be healthy generally, they must remain active. A range of senior-friendly physical activities that support cardiovascular health, strength, flexibility, and balance are covered in this chapter. Promoting regular exercise improves mental and emotional health in addition to physical health.

1. **Walking and Brisk Walking:** Emphasize the advantages of walking for elderly people. Promote brisk walking as an easy-to-use yet powerful technique to preserve joint flexibility, elevate mood, and improve cardiovascular health.

2. **Chair Exercises:** Provide an overview of chair exercises. Seniors with mobility issues can benefit from sitting exercises, which help them become more flexible and stronger.

3. **Water Aerobics:** Examine the advantages of participating in water aerobics. This low-impact exercise is appropriate for seniors with different levels of fitness because it is easy on the joints and provides resistance for strength training.

4. **Yoga for Seniors:** Encourage senior yoga. Stress has advantages for stress relief, balance, and flexibility.

Seniors with varying needs and skills can select from a variety of modified yoga poses.

5. Tai Chi: Tai Chi is a soft, flowing kind of exercise. This age-old technique is especially helpful for elders since it improves balance, coordination, and mental focus.

6. Resistance Band Workouts: Include exercises with resistance bands. These are good for seniors who want to increase muscle tone since they offer resistance for strength training without requiring large weights.

7. Senior-Friendly Dance Lessons: Examine dance lessons that are appropriate for seniors. Dancing is a fun and social activity for seniors to stay active. It might be ballroom, line, or dance-based health classes.

8. Gardening and Yard Work: Emphasize the health advantages of yard work and gardening. These exercises work different muscle groups, increase flexibility, and give you a sense of achievement.

9. Golfing: Seniors who take pleasure in outdoor activities should be encouraged to play golf. Golf enhances social contact and offers mild aerobic activity, both of which are beneficial to general wellbeing.

10. Cycling: Talk about the advantages of cycling. Seniors who want to strengthen their legs and cardiovascular systems can select between stationary bikes and regular bicycles.

11. Senior Fitness Classes: Look into senior fitness programs offered by nearby gyms or community centers. The particular requirements and preferences of senior citizens are the focus of these classes.

12. Senior Pilates: Present Pilates as a low-impact workout. Pilates is appropriate for seniors who want to increase their general body stability since it emphasizes core strength, flexibility, and balance.

13. Gentle Stretching Practice: Encourage the practice of gentle stretching. Seniors can preserve their mobility and avoid stiffness by engaging in stretching exercises that improve their flexibility and joint range of motion.

14. Balance exercises: Make sure to incorporate these. Simple exercises that improve stability and lower the chance of falling include heel-to-toe walking, standing on one leg, and using balance boards.

15. Mind-Body Practices: Place special emphasis on mind-body techniques like deep breathing and meditation. Stress reduction, brain clarity, and general emotional well-being are all enhanced by these exercises.

Holistic Approaches to Enhance Overall Well-being for Seniors

In order to achieve comprehensive well-being, one must attend to one's mental, emotional, and physical well-being. This chapter delves into a variety of holistic approaches specifically designed for senior citizens, promoting an all-encompassing strategy to improve their general well-being.

1. "Mentality Meditation: Give a brief explanation of mindfulness meditation. Mindfulness techniques can help seniors feel less stressed, more focused, and more emotionally healthy.

2. Soft Yoga and Stretching: Give special attention to soft yoga and stretching. Engaging in these activities fosters a complete mind-body connection by promoting both physical and mental calm.

3. Outdoor Activities and Nature Hikes: Promote outdoor activities and nature hikes. It has been demonstrated that spending time in nature improves mental health by lowering stress and fostering serenity.

4. Creativity and Art Sessions: Examine creative and art sessions. Painting or creating are examples of artistic endeavors that give people a creative outlet and improve their emotional health.

5. Community Involvement and Social Engagement: Stress the value of social involvement. Seniors can improve their quality of life by participating in social activities and maintaining relationships with friends, family, and the community.

6. Holistic Nutrition Seminars: Provide information about seminars on holistic nutrition. Seniors who want to make holistic dietary decisions might adopt a more informed perspective by learning about the relationship between nutrition, general health, and well-being.

7. Treatment and Conventional Chinese Medicine: Examine treatment with acupuncture and conventional Chinese medicine. These holistic methods can help the body achieve equilibrium and manage a range of health issues.

8. Massage Therapy and Bodywork: Talk about the advantages of bodywork and massage therapy. In addition to promoting physical relaxation, these activities help lower stress and improve emotional health in general.

9. Pranayama and Breathing Exercises: Instruct students in pranayama and breathing exercises. Seniors who want to improve lung function, lower stress levels, and foster mental clarity should practice controlled breathing exercises.

10. Activities for Cognitive Stimulation: Place a focus on activities for cognitive stimulation. Playing games, solving puzzles, or continuing education can improve cognitive function in general and mental acuity.

11. Essential Oils and Aromatherapy: Explain the use of essential oils and aromatherapy. Scents can have a beneficial effect on mood and relaxation, giving elders a comprehensive approach to emotional health.

12. Listening Sessions and Music Therapy: Encourage listening sessions and music therapy. Positive feelings, stress reduction, and improved emotional and mental health can all be achieved through music listening.

13. Energy Healing Techniques: Learn about energy healing techniques. Energy-based therapies such as Qi Gong, Reiki, and others can help to create harmony and balance in both the body and the mind.

14. Activities with a Purpose and Volunteering:
Promote activities with a purpose and volunteer. Taking
part in endeavors that enhance the welfare of others can
provide one with a feeling of direction and satisfaction.

15. Adequate Sleep Hygiene Practices: Highlight how
crucial it is to follow appropriate sleep hygiene
procedures. A good night's sleep is crucial for mental and
physical recovery and for maintaining general wellbeing.

CONCLUSION

We've discovered a wealth of information in this investigation into a low-salt lifestyle designed specifically for seniors that goes beyond the traditional concept of dietary limitations. This journey has fundamentally been about empowering seniors by providing them with the knowledge they need to make decisions that align with their health goals. The talk underscores that leading a low-salt lifestyle is not a restriction but rather a means to an active and satisfying old age, from understanding food labels to commemorating significant occasions.

A lighthouse of culinary innovation appeared, showing the way to tasty and fulfilling meals without sacrificing health objectives. Seniors were encouraged to use different herbs, spices, and culinary methods, converting the kitchen into a happy and creative place. This culinary dimension celebrates the art of living, where the search for well-being and the joy of indulging in a well-prepared meal are intertwined. It goes beyond simply cutting back on sodium intake.

This discourse has been braided throughout the social fabric of well-being. The value of social relationships in the health journey is emphasized with techniques for interacting with loved ones during milestone celebrations, navigating restaurant menus, and conveying dietary preferences. A community that is encouraging and understanding can be a great ally for seniors navigating the triad of making health-conscious decisions and participating in social activities. This talk has laid the groundwork for a story of strength, resiliency, and the happy pursuit of health and happiness in one's golden years in the overall fabric of physical, mental, and emotional well-being.

www.ingramcontent.com/pod-product-compliance
Lightning Source LLC
Chambersburg PA
CBHW070904260726

48661CB00004B/1583